T0129276

You Won't Learn This
in Massage School

You Won't Learn This in Massage School

Cynthia Boccuti, LMT

authorHOUSE®

AuthorHouse™
1663 Liberty Drive
Bloomington, IN 47403
www.authorhouse.com
Phone: 1-800-839-8640

Published by AuthorHouse   01/16/2013

ISBN: 978-1-4817-0556-1 (sc)
ISBN: 978-1-4817-0555-4 (e)

Library of Congress Control Number: 2013900477

Any people depicted in stock imagery provided by Thinkstock are models,
and such images are being used for illustrative purposes only.
Certain stock imagery © Thinkstock.

This book is printed on acid-free paper.

I have my husband, Tony, to thank for being the most supportive of my career change. From day one he never wavered and has always been my biggest fan. I love him for being my center and my sounding board. I also am thrilled to have had massage-addicted family and friends, most notably my daughter Melissa and best friend Dani, who have always been ready to try the newest technique or spa treatment. You all have encouraged me and allowed me to become who I am as a person and a therapist.

This is also for all the clients during all my years of working in this wonderful field. They have each brought something unique to the (massage) table and taught me some things that I hope to share with as many readers as I can.

Thank you from the bottom of my heart.

CONTENTS

Foreword

There are things in life that must be experienced. Experience is our best teacher but sometimes learning from others experiences can be a great learning tool also. Talking with people and even more importantly, listening to what they have to say are the most important experiences. If you're lucky enough or smart enough you will have the opportunity to do this repeatedly with your clients for many years.

Over the 17 years in self-employed practice, I have had my share of those moments. When it's all said and done, I have learned so much about the human body and mind that I should already have my sociology degree.

If I'm to share with you any of my stories, I would want you to understand that this book is less about making tens of thousands of dollars than it is about the process of making tens of thousands of clients happy.

When I began this career in massage, a wise woman once told me and I quote, "Cyndi, it's not about the money." I thought surely it wasn't for her. She had a healthy, established clientele and well, I was just starting out and had NONE. For me, in those days, it was ALL about the money. I had a young child, a mortgage, expenses and so forth. With mounting bills and little money in the bank to start this new career, I had a really hard time embracing her concept. It just seemed so unreasonable to me. I wanted to just make the money to do my part of raising income for my family. I had a lot to learn.

The information found in this book is helpful in adopting a mindset and practices you can use to be successful and become a better therapist. This is with the benefit of a client's perspective and a massage therapist's experience. Being successful doesn't mean only having book smarts. While that is inherently important, there are components to this career that when honed, can position you as being the best massage therapist your clients will ever experience. It's imperative to have good hands, good knowledge of the body, and a good physiology background. That should be fairly evident. You need to listen carefully. The basics you learn in massage school. The lessons you learn beyond graduation from your school will make that difference.

I will also share some humorous stories and anecdotes to help illustrate my points. These stories don't necessarily help your clients directly but will help you deal WITH them.

You won't learn this in school. There are no credits courses for this knowledge and you can't really place a value on it, except for what this book just cost you. But I promise, I will make it as enjoyable and helpful as possible.

I hope you have fun learning about your field of massage and the great people you will come to appreciate as your clients.

Session One
WHAT'S ON THAT INTAKE FORM AGAIN?

Have you ever wondered about when you visit your doctor's office and fill out those health forms? Do the employees or assistants even look at what you just answered? Sometimes it seems like they just ask you the same questions when you go back to the exam room rather than take a peek at what you just spent 15 minutes writing down. Sometimes they may be double-checking with you and that's fine but it does get you wondering about how much attention they are paying to your records.

If a client takes the time to get out their doctor's phone numbers and write down their medications for us, the least we can do is scan the form. But, if we're better than average, we will notice smaller bits of information like their birthday, if they've had previous massages, where they live and so on.

Not only do these serve as talking points that make them feel like we care and it gives us additional information to help us understand our client's goals while they're on the table.

I couldn't tell you how many times I've had a surprised look and a THANK YOU from them because I noticed their birthday was that day, or is approaching. It takes people off guard that we notice something seemingly insignificant but see it as important to them. It also can tell us that it might be stressful turning the big 4-0 or some other milestone birthday. Where they live might offer clues about tree allergies or road work that they've had to deal with. All extra stressors that they bring to the massage.

What kind of occupation do they have? Body mechanics and physical demands, travel time, computer work, phone calls, etcetera. It matters. . . a lot.

If your new client has had massage, whether frequent or not, what did they like or dislike about it? Replicate what they like, using your own style but definitely don't repeat the things that gave them reason to search out another therapist. Remember that's possibly why they are seeing you for the first time.

You want them to return so pay attention to verbal and non-verbal information.

So how much time does all this extra attention cost you? It takes about 3 minutes to make an impact on someone you expect will love your hands and your work enough to make a commitment to their health by returning. Total time for the intake may be 5-10 minutes and you've already got them poised to relax or at least able to communicate with you if the work requires more client input. This is time well spent in my book.

After the intake form we want to direct them to the massage room. On occasion, we may have a 'chatty' client. There are tricks to getting them into the massage room and on the table on time. If they have a lot of health issues, it's important to spend extra time discussing those topics so you are sure that there are no contraindications. In general though, non verbal clues will do the trick. Begin by walking toward the massage room or a wave of your hand so as to indicate they should follow you. Either or both of these is usually effective. For others you may need to say it outright, "Well let's get you ready so we can start close to your appointment time." Be upfront but not obnoxious.

You may have a client immediately after them but they don't know that and frankly some people just lose track of time. They can be so sociable. So take the lead and they'll probably follow. Be sure to tell them you'll be ready for them in a moment so they don't dawdle.

Session Two
HOW TO LISTEN~

"Oh, I didn't put that on the form"

When my daughter was a teenager, I heard somewhere that the best way to learn what is important to a teen or going on in their lives is while driving in the car because they don't have to make eye contact. It's funny how that always seemed true. When in the massage room, the same principle seems to apply.

When people aren't face down on the table all kinds of information just comes billowing forth. It may be inadvertent, but somehow while you massage people they remember things. You'll hear comments like, 'When I was in that car accident last week', 'I had surgery on my shoulder last year.', 'My doctor wants me to see a specialist.' It can go on and on like that. It's amazing how that information was missing on the health intake form.

You may learn about some important factors that have a bearing on how you'll proceed with your session. You'll find out soon enough that going with the flow is paramount. Adjusting your strokes, your pressure or where you'll spend a greater amount of time based on the new information should be fluid.

If you notice scars, stab wounds from arthroscopic surgery or that their joints don't have full range of motion, feel free to question the client. You can't read minds and rather than cause pain or injury, simply ask.

They should be able to fill in the blanks for you. In fact, they may think that information is insignificant when it could be important enough to require an adjustment to the massage techniques.

I learned one day while massaging a gentleman, that he couldn't flex his fingers and wrist well on one side. When I questioned him in a curious tone about it he told me it was the result of being in several motorcycle accidents years before and as it turned out, he was lucky to be alive. Limited range of motion for him was a non-issue. He had his life. Well, that never showed up on the intake health form. Needless to say, I adjusted the hand and arm massage to accommodate his range of motion based on this new information.

If someone has scars that they don't mention, go ahead and do cross fiber friction on them if you feel scar tissue build up. You can also share with them what you're doing and they'll know you are addressing an area they didn't realize would matter because it hadn't become bothersome yet. It's acceptable to ask why they have them and in doing that you might uncover more information. You don't really want to be chatty but asking these kinds of questions could be important.

Ask the questions. No one expects you to know it all. I ask all the time about some of the new medicines that clients write on my intake forms. I certainly am not the Physician's Desk Reference book with all the possible prescription drugs out there on the market. Medicine evolves and new drugs are being prescribed. Don't assume that it's unimportant. You might find that they are on anti-depressants, anti-rejection medicines or psych drugs. Does your client have an internal pacemaker or defibrillator? How should you handle that? You may find that it's quite an interesting field with all the different issues that people bring to the massage office and that we have as a whole population. These are just some of the situations we face in this field. Also because it's considered alternative, we often hear about different ways of treating health issues. Clients may seek energy work, homeopathic treatment, colonics, and nutritional or dietary changes to address their needs. So not only do we find it necessary to understand the medical model, we need to be aware of complementary care approaches.

We can't be experts in all aspects of the health field but that is often times what is so compelling about what we do. We continually expand our horizons by listening to the clients who encourage us to be educated about new treatments.

It's essential to have an awareness of their mental and physical health especially as it relates to their massage.

Not surprisingly, people love to talk about themselves. Even after years of having a massage practice, there will still be many issues that will arise and that you'll learn from. True edification.

Ultimately, you are the professional. In your clients' opinions, you are the expert in your field, whether you have a week of experience or years. Clients don't usually differentiate. They want the best every time and you can give that to them if you are aware and if you care to be improve on all phases of your career.

Session Three
WIGS AND THINGS~

Dealing with hairy situations

I have had my share of cancer patients but one day I was a bit surprised while massaging the scalp of one lady. It just didn't feel quite like other scalps so I paid a little closer attention and realized that she was wearing a wig. Understanding by her reluctance to share this with me, I did not mention it to her. Perhaps baldness or thinning hair was an issue for her and she felt ill at ease in mentioning it to me. Perhaps it was just a simple change in fashion for her. That could also be a possibility.

Rather than massage the wig any longer, I spent more time on her facial muscles, ears and sub occipital area. Even after the massage, there was no mention of her wearing a wig so I left it as a personal choice on her part to not disclose that to me. There were no other indicators or information on her intake health sheet that would have left me a good reason to question her further about the wig.

At that point, it was just a matter of respect for her privacy.

Still, there are times when patients who are being treated for cancer or who are recovering from treatments have little or no hair. You'll probably be aware of this since it would be covered on the intake form. People who have been recently treated with chemotherapy have a port and they'll show you where it's located on their chest. Feel free to ask if they'd like to remove the wig or scarf so that you can massage their scalp. Interestingly enough, they'll probably jump at it. For a lot of cancer patients, no one touches their heads and it always feels so good to have your head massaged. If they decline, it is also okay, but in my experience, it's always been something they enjoyed.

I don't know why but some of the yummiest parts of our bodies to have massaged are the endpoints. Head, hands and feet feel so good when they are touched and massaged. So go for it. They'll love every minute of it. You'll want to give them extra time after the massage session to get their 'look' back in order before exiting your office.

Another challenge we face is the person who has excessive hair. You will most likely come across this, I promise. One of the easiest ways to work on someone who has a lot of hair is to use oil or gel. Creams can often times clump or knot the hair on the legs or their backs. Lotions are ineffective also. I've learned that the thicker the lubricant, the more trouble it's going to be in this situation.

You may or may not encounter clients who have had organ transplants. During one of my in home visits, my client shared with me that before his heart transplant and before taking anti-rejection medications, he was completely bald and had very little body hair. It was verified by his family members too because I had never heard of that kind of a response to medication. What a strange reaction, I thought. But sure enough, they showed me photos of him pre and post surgery and follow ups and there was a striking change. I was amazed that his arm, leg and back hair was so thick that I wondered if I would be able to massage him without pulling his hair whereby making the session less than relaxing. He was always pleased with his sessions so I may have just been overly sensitive to the situation. The unscented oil worked best in his case.

On a different note, I once had a client who had a colostomy bag. This person was very comfortable with sharing this news with me and was able to make me at ease as well. It was something that he had for years so his ability to make it a normal topic of conversation was impressive. Frankly, I think that's why I responded without hesitation or anxiety about how to handle or deal with the bag during the massage.

Some clients may also have hearing aids to remove. If they do not use them during the massage, you may want to use some tactile cues to get their attention by a shoulder tap or some other means. Once they know you're trying to speak to them, they may be able to read your lips or watch your hand gestures to understand what you're trying to communicate. Sometimes we get to be creative in communicating. Eventually thinking outside the box will become normal.

Even on unimpaired clients, I always touch the arm or leg to let them know where I will be working next. It serves as notice that they can relax that area and it also prevents them from jumping as you go from limb to limb. Sometimes they lose track of where you are if you remove your hands too frequently. The massage can seem broken up or choppy. I make it a practice to keep contact as much as possible to keep the flow.

Session Four
WEIGHTY ISSUES

From time to time, you will encounter someone who is excessively overweight. It's sometimes emotional for them to be undressed in front of therapists and it's a serious issue. Some clients are reluctant to get massage because they are uncomfortable with their weight. Know your table and products. That's good, common sense on any given day. Some times it becomes more important when you need to put someone at ease and it's as simple as explaining what you know about the equipment you use.

As a therapist you see people of different shapes and sizes all the time but have no idea what their lives are like or the baggage that they carry. One of the kindest things we can do as people is to not judge too critically.

The Golden Rule: treat others as you would have them treat you. This is really the best way to approach everyone.

I have had clients come to the office and tell me that they'd like to bring their significant other or spouse in to the office for a massage but that person is overweight and worries that the table may break. Seriously. That has happened and not just once in my career.

Now as I've said before, it's important to know your products. I knew the static weight that my table could withstand and assured my client that their person would not break my table unless they jumped up and down on it. I wanted to interject a little levity to the conversation but did not diminish the seriousness of their concerns. I thought there was no way anyone could be THAT overweight so as to hurt themselves while on the table or even break it. Months after that conversation, that very person came in for a massage and to be frank was quite large but had an equally large heart. Very personable, really intelligent and very caring.

I could see what my client loved about this person and why they wanted to share massage experiences with them. Inside each of us is the very essence of who we are and regardless of the external size. It's the stuff that makes us who we are that always shows through. It's nice to know that we don't all get judged wholly on our external appearances. We all have bad days but we'd like to think that there is more to us than just what someone sees.

Talk with people as if they are average Joe's. Find out what they like about massage and if they've had massages before. If a skinny person walked in the door that's what you'd do. So why treat a larger person any differently? Ask about their jobs, body mechanics, etc. Don't make it about weight. If they verbalize concern about the table breaking or falling off the side of the table, be reassuring. For them, it's a very real concern and they will likely be serious about this with you.

Let them know that you wouldn't want anyone to fall or have reservations while being massaged. The session should be about them relaxing and free from concern. Basically, walk them through the process when it's time to turn over.

While massaging someone of size be sure to work those muscles thoroughly. Think of it this way, those muscles work harder to support and move limbs than on a small-framed person. In a sense, heavier people may actually need the petrissage more.

Larger women in general tend to feel less sexy, so be considerate. Curves are coming back in style but for a large portion of society, curves mean fat. Fat means ugly; you get the idea. It's not our job to make them feel pretty or handsome but it is our job to make them relax. It's all part of the same goal. This is where the mind body connection comes into play.

Here are some other considerations. Perhaps your overweight client has had an abusive past and eating was a defense mechanism. It could be a result of heredity that some people are predisposed to carry more weight than others. Perhaps your client is in the process of having bariatric surgery and is currently morbidly obese but looking to be healthier after surgery. The point is that we are all different and bring those differences to the massage office. There are layers to people and they need to be seen for who they are, not how much they are. Genuineness makes a clear difference in whether you see them for a second session. That's food for thought.

Session Five
So That's What Aromatherapy Is For~

Aromatherapy is a wonderful treat to the senses and is intended to bring out particular responses in the client's limbic system. Oils are extracts of roots and leaves of plants that cause reactions in the body when inhaled, added to steam or carrier oils for application. It is often times an important addition to the session enabling the client to relax at a different level.

One additional use for aromatherapy is just to cover some unpleasant odors. I wouldn't use the expensive essential oils for the latter; I would use something a little less refined but will still have do the trick.

Body odor is not pleasant and more often than not, the person with the offending scent, interestingly enough, is blissfully unaware. They are accustomed to their own smells. We are all like that. Hopefully as therapists, we are more aware of what we bring to the table as well and the spacial relationship that exists between the position of the client and our own bodies, if you know what I mean. Alas, as their therapist, you can get a schnoz-full at times.

There is no easy way to get away from someone whose hygiene is somewhat challenging. Range of motion for their arms may awaken the beast. Creative breathing, some scented oils or creams help mask the offending armpit odor but you'll want to return the arm to it's original position sooner than later.

Feet present an easier situation. We can always work through the sheets when it's necessary and the clients don't seem to think anything of it. Perhaps people are funny about their feet because they know they've worn shoes all day and most people have stinky feet after a day of work. There are also some really great foot balms or creams on the market that use peppermint oils. These creams are great for making feet tingle and feel refreshed.

Go ahead and let your client know that your are giving them an extra treat for their feet. It's so magnanimous of you. You're always looking for ways to make your client's visit a little more special. It's tip worthy, trust me, but you're also benefitting from less foot odor or bacteria.

Different smelly situations occur often enough. I could not tell you how many times I've had clients pass gas, toot or what have you. Funny enough, it happens when you are focusing on the strokes and how the muscles are responding, the music is quiet, perhaps the water fountain is gurgling in the background and the client is utterly relaxed and just zoning off and all of a sudden. PFFTTT!!!

You jump cause you're startled out of your own zone. You want to laugh, inside of course, because you just didn't expect it. Then there it is, undeniable and loud. Usually it's accompanied by a smell. What do you do? Turn your head and breathe. If you can reach for some aromatherapy scents, quickly place a drop or spritz quietly in the air to offset the unpleasantness. A small amount is usually sufficient and you will want to do this in a way that you don't offend your client either. I'm sure they are either glad you took control in masking what they could be potentially embarrassed about. When clients relax, this happens but if they say anything to you, you can put them at ease by making light of it and tell them that you were just getting them too relaxed. If you assume responsibility for that, they'll appreciate it. But again, they'll probably like the extra scent in the room during their massage. Tip worthy?

Part of the relaxation process involves the parasympathetic nervous system. It's that rest and digest mode that we know about. So many clients will have stomach gurgling or growling and the first thing they do is to hold their stomach. They don't realize that it's very common during a massage.

Some of that growling may be due to hunger but for a lot of people it means that they are relaxing. That's what we want to hear. You can reassure them that it's perfectly normal and fine.

Frankly, it could happen on the other end too. Think about it. As therapists we'd like to think we'll never have our stomachs gurgle, pass gas or have bad breath but sometimes it happens.

Try your best to be clean and prepared for sessions. Use your best judgement.

In addition to smells and sounds, there is body fluid. Drool, in particular . . . . The very first time I learned about drool is embedded in my mind. At the time, I was glad that my client was relaxed enough to nod off but I was unaware of the dark side to that relaxation until I had him turn onto his back. I should have looked at the stool that was beneath the face piece. Should. Have. Looked. Once the client was settled in the new position, I pulled the stool out to sit and SPLASH DOWN.

I knew immediately what happened but I could not react. It would have been wrong to do so because it would have embarrassed the client. I just lifted and set a hand towel down on the stool so that I could continue without my client being any wiser to the situation.

It's comical when I think about it now but that was a tough one.

Session Six
STIFLE IT~

It happens to all of us at some point. You don't plan to have a reaction to dust, a client's perfume or whatever the trigger is. You will have to sneeze. The problem is that you don't want to spread germs or give your client the idea that you can just spray the room with your sneeze and it's all supposed to be okay.

What do you do? How can you stop something like that? Can you? Why yes you can.

I don't recall exactly how it came to me but it's tried and true and is effective. I developed seasonal allergies as I got older and had to find a solution to this annoying little occurrence while I was in the massage room.

Sneezes are important to body functions so stifling one is not necessarily what you'd want to do all the time but in this instance, it's fine. Sneezing allows the body to rid itself of unwanted bacteria and irritants. It has a purpose in maintaining our health.

Here's my trick:

When you can feel a sneeze coming on, pinch the bridge of your nose just where it goes from cartilage to nasal flaps so that your nose is closed. You may need to go through the pseudo-motion of the sneeze with your mouth open but nothing else really happens. It actually will suppress the sneeze. You have to let your body go through it's cycle to kind of fool it.

All the while, your hand is on the client. You can continue to massage and they are none the wiser. no sneeze, no concern about germs. As long as you aren't putting your fingers in your nose or at the entrance to your nose, you should be fine but to be on the safe side, tissues could be handy in your room and easily discarded without an issue. Also you may have one of those alcohol hand sanitizing gel pumps near by. As for the client, though, their session was uninterrupted and smooth.

Session Seven
WHEN WOULD YOU LIKE TO RESCHEDULE?

How to rebook clients

Easily enough, all you need to do is ask when and not 'if' they'd like to put something on the calendar. I usually just lead with, "Would you like to schedule something for next month or would you rather email me when you know what your schedule looks like?" Sometimes I ask "Should we see what next month looks like for you?" "Take your cues from their body language throughout the time you've just spent with them. You may want to suggest something sooner depending on what you learn in their first session with you. If a quick follow up session would help them, make that suggestion. Sometimes clients ask when we would suggest they return. Remembering that your are the experienced therapist, it's just fine to assist with those decisions. When the question or suggestion of making another appointment is posed from a place of genuine care for them, it's a positive experience.

You want to present yourself as a self-assured therapist yet relaxed in knowing that you are available for them. You never want to seem over-zealous or insistent that they rebook immediately. Not everyone responds well to that. I have seen the semi hard sell backfire like crazy on some therapists. They may think that it comes across as confident but some clients really prefer to call when THEY feel like it. They don't want that nudge at all. So be open to how your clients operate. Everyone is different and it is in no way a reflection of your massage. Some of my best and most loyal clients NEVER make an appointment for the next session but they call religiously month after month for many years. That works for them and for me, too.

One thing to note is that if people tell you that their lives are crazy and super busy, you can phrase it to them as though this is an important part of making their life a bit less stressful.

Sometimes having a date and time on the calendar in advance allows them to look forward to some de-stressing and physical stress relief. It becomes a good appointment to have on their calendar. Whatever they choose to do has to be what works for them. Too much urging is not going to persuade them. I will often times suggest that if it's on the calendar, they know that the time is theirs and they can always have the option to call to cancel 24 hours ahead, to reschedule or cancel if need be. If they choose to wait, that time may not be available later. Again, it has to be their choice.

Session Eight
OPTIMIZING GIFT CARDS

Prior to holidays like Christmas, Mother'sDay and Father's day, Valentine's Day and so on, I regularly put signs up in my office letting them know that I sell gift cards. The best places to post are bathrooms and wherever you have your clients pay for their sessions or rebook appointments. Usually it's because they are in one place for a few minutes and have time to look around. That's the whole premise of impulse buying at the supermarkets. Put reminders where people spend the most time. Right next to that sign be sure that they also see the 'credit cards accepted' signs, too. After all, it should be a simple and convenient purchase for them.

I love selling gift cards to my clients. It means that they trust me to take care of the people they like. It means they value what I do and they're willing to share me with people they know. I have made the post card size cards out the old-fashioned way forever and I actually prefer it. The hand-written cards can be personalized rather than those credit type style of cards. I put the expiration date clearly on it and almost never have problems with people redeeming them.

The newer version of debit style cards works well but the older version is just my preference. There are advantages and disadvantages to both styles so research is always a good idea whichever you choose to use.

One advantage to clients getting the debit style is that if it's lost they can recover it sometimes. Also as time expires, there is no debate about it's value. There is a company that will charge a processing fee and that is deducted from the card if it is inactive or has not been used beyond a certain date which I believe is usually two years. That's something to check on wherever you practice massage.

The paper gift card stands out because it doesn't get mixed in with the usual cards in a wallet or purse. The post card size seems popular too.

Over the years, I realize that clients for the most part know what the gift recipient likes and will purchase it just like that, per treatment. Another option is to make it out for a specific dollar amount. This seems to be less stressful for the purchaser and gives flexibility to the recipient if you offer different spa treatments or massage add-on packages.

When gifts are given specifying a dollar amount, clients are more apt to come in more than once to experience your massage because they have value left on the gift card. As a therapist, it presents an additional opportunity to retain them as long term clients because they get to know you better. You are better able to work within their tolerances because you will get to know them better also. When you learn about your client's preferences or tolerances with pressure and so on, it makes the experience so much better.

In an effort to make paying for successive treatments simple, credit and debit machines can increase your finances. It's convenient for the clients or gift card purchasers. People love to use plastic and will worry about paying it off their charges later but the sales will increase more by offering it. The small fee you pay to the processing company will definitely be offset by the amount of money you'll bring in with one.

Credit card merchant companies differ greatly and flexibility is important so do your due diligence if you decide to go that route. There can be significant differences in how they charge you as the business and they should be motivated to get your processing business.

There are so many different types of terminals available that it doesn't matter if you are mobile or in one centralized location, there is every reason to use this option. Do some research with the massage association affiliates.

There are deals and discounts out there. You just need to tap into that resource.

Session Nine
IT'S T TIME~

How to weed out the late clients, the no-shows and the deal-makers.

It can be a challenge when clients are habitually late, forgetful of their appointment times or just down right inconsiderate and cancel with little time for you to book anyone else in their slot. Of all the wonderful things that come with being a massage therapist, this one is the disadvantage and the toughest, I think.

We can put up signs, make the clients sign a paper that states the fees for missed appointments and similar policies, but enforcing them is a whole other ball game. Clients need to understand that the time they have reserved for their massage is the time that they should be on the table, not just arriving and then using the facilities, then turning off the phone and chatting with you. It's Table Time. T-TIME.

On one hand, we want all the clients we can get. We like what we do, we want to make money doing it so we put up with a certain amount of difficult people in order to achieve those goals. On the other hand, we don't want to turn people away.

At some point, though, there is a reason to remind them of those rules and why they are important. At some point there is a reason to start enforcing the policy, It's a tough decision and the response may not be received well, but I promise you that one of two things will happen in the end. Firstly, they will pay and let you know they aren't happy about it. To which you kindly defer to the posted signs and the signed paper you had from their first visit. They will either pay and return and never make the mistake of missing an appointment again or they will pay and not return. I have learned over the years that if they don't return because they don't like that policy then it's probably best to not have them as clients. They are problematic and they are disrespectful. Frankly do you really want to keep them on as clients if they don't respect your time or the time of other clients?

Session Ten
DO I HAVE TO
ANSWER THAT?

It's a funny business

Now that licensing is in full swing nationwide, we need to be professional all the time. There is no sliding by; no seeing clients without first having all the info necessary to ensure a safe and effective massage session. We therapists need to be certain we have all the health information before we lay hands on anyone. It's just a prudent course of action. How we dress; the way we present ourselves; the questions we ask; how we speak and so on speaks volumes about our practice and who we are personally. So be clear about your intentions and body mechanics when you greet a new client. It helps to have items around such as diplomas and ethics rules posted on your wall somewhere which can be subtle but make an impact. If you wear a uniform or a shirt with the business name on it, that helps deter the undesirable people.

I've also noticed that if women are frequent clients in the office, men get the idea without having to make the wrong guess about your establishment.

Subtle clues should be all you need to get the point across to them. If it isn't and they ask vague questions like "what do I get in the hour?" simply ask them if they can be more specific. Always put the ball in their court because you never know that they are searching for a happy ending. They may honestly not know what is covered in a session. So don't presume; just ask them to be more clear. That will almost always take care of the situation.

Years ago when massage therapy wasn't so mainstream, there was the prevalent idea that all massage therapists were working for massage parlors and gave a little extra at the end of the massage. While my office was not like that, it didn't stop the occasional assumption on the part of some walk-in clients.

When I first opened my office, I expected to get my fair share of those kinds of clients but, frankly, I didn't really have TOO many. There were a few. One that stands out though was a man who walked in and asked if I had time to see him. Since the office was new to the area and my day was fairly light, I didn't think it wise to say no to anyone. I had the time that day, so I said I had time for a massage.

As he walked further into the office, about 5 feet, I reached for my intake form and clipboard and proceeded to ask him to fill it out. Immediately, the expression on his face changed to surprise and then concern. He asked if he had to fill it out. I was clear in telling him it was absolutely necessary.

He began to back up while explaining to me that he left his glasses in the car. (side note: he had not parked anywhere near the office) He said he'd be right back and I told him it would be no problem for me to just read off the questions on this one page form so that he could answer them. He insisted that he'd rather just get his glasses and he'd be right back. He explained that he just lived down the street but since I live directly across from my home on a fairly quiet street and know my neighbors quite well, I just knew it was a story that he was telling me. You can see where this is going, I'm sure. I then realized, by his reaction, what was going on so I pressed him to just answer what he could. It was only a health form after all. He said, no, that's okay. If the whole situation lasted 2 minutes it was forever for him. I think he was backing out of the office through out the entire exchange. I laughed to myself.

I was a bit miffed too because I really wanted to be accepted as a legitimate massage therapist in my new office and didn't want THAT kind of clientele. I wanted it to be clear that I was not running a massage parlor.

In all the years I have practiced, I have only been propositioned once and I was so irritated by it. The client was quietly moaning as some people do but almost gyrating on the table during the initial part of the massage helped me realize what was going on. At first I thought it just felt good and he needed the work. Then he continued with remarks that were inappropriate. The client was verbally persistent. I think what I was most disturbed by was that he assumed that he could convince me that it was the right thing to do. I should have just ended the massage as soon as all that started but I really believed that I could just explain that the 'extras' were not going to happen and that he would discontinue his efforts. Still he went on and told me It was "about taking care of business". That last comment did it for me. I was emphatic when I told him the session was over and he could pay me for the whole session before he left. I also told him that he was banned from the office and if he was to approach me or any other therapist in my office, we would be calling the police.

I can imagine for male therapists, there are similar situations with female clients coming on to them but I can't really speak to that. The same rules apply though. Be professional; be clear and if you have done that, you have done your best to give show them there is no 'funny business' at your establishment. It can take you by surprise when it happens though. I almost wish that I had ended the session earlier in the exchange.

The best thing you can do is to be very clear in your purpose as a therapist whether the person is standing in front of you or on the phone asking these very same questions. I can tell you that when confronted with this kind of client, it was difficult to keep my emotions in check. I wanted to be disgusted and angry but I knew that I had to remain calm and professional. It was a challenge but I found that being straightforward and clearly professional was the best approach.

Assumptions may be made anyway but it won't be because you have misrepresented yourself.

Session Eleven
PICKY, PICKY

When I worked in a chiropractic office right after graduation, I was their employee and had no control over who I would see. It was the chiropractor's decision to send people on for massage and my responsibility to tend to the areas that would complement the adjustment.

Most people were fairly compliant with the work but there was one woman who I just thought I'd never please. She would complain to the chiropractor about how one thing or another that bothered her. He would in turn relay it to me. I expect to do my best so this was a frustrating experience. If it wasn't pressure, it was temperature, don't do that, do this. It went on for weeks. I couldn't seem to figure out how to make the massage work for her or me. As therapists we always strive to do the best for the patient or client.

So I figuratively stepped back from it for a bit one day, assessed the situation pragmatically and formulated a plan for her next session. I decided that because she was an educator at the collegiate level, communicating with her about each stroke and it's purpose might work well. If she could tell me what pressure was comfortable, then I would maintain it. As it turned out, this was perfect.

As an educator at a nearby university, she was very cerebral and questioned everything. It wasn't because she mistrusted my work, it was because she had a need to understand.

Effective communication between us and an understanding of the session's goals was exactly what she expected. It was something I could easily do, too.

Clients bring different personalities, history and preferences to the table and paying attention to those clues, while sometimes subtle, can improve you as a person and therapist. Personal and professional edification comes in many forms. It takes years to hone those skills.

It is said that if you want to work with someone, learn how they operate. If they're visual, use those visual terms but if they're thinkers then work with them from that point of view. Some people use terms like, "I see what you're saying" or "I hear you" because they function on a visual or auditory level. Adapting to your client helps both of you. Sometimes it takes a little investigation or trial and error but then again, you may just luck out.

Session Twelve
DIZZY, OLD PEOPLE

There are times when the elderly can just out and out surprise you with the things they say or do. Maybe when we get to a certain age, there is less of a filter or people just don't care to stand on protocol anymore. I'm talking about those folks over the age of 75 or so. I am really not sure what it is about this demographic but they have a peculiar way of quickly undressing while you're still showing them to the room or while explaining what you want them to do so as to make them comfortable in the room. Then there is the extreme situation when they just pull the sheets away to show you a mole in an area that doesn't see the sun often. They are adamant that you see it too. This has happened only on a rare occasion but with my women clients more frequently than men. Even so, it's just as surprising when it happens and comical when you think about it later.

The only proper thing you should do is tell them to contact their doctor if it's a health issue. Be as matter-of-fact as possible when telling them that you see what they are showing you but it's out of your scope of practice to address the issue. Phrase it however you feel is appropriate for the situation. No one wants to embarrass the client or feel embarrassed by being asked. So being discreet, professional and tactful is key.

On a more serious and literal note, as our clients age there is a predisposition toward dizziness that occurs when they try to get up from the table too quickly. Occasionally it is due to medications that they're taking but more often than not, it's advancing age. Head rushes can lead to clients succumbing to the perils of gravity. A simple word of caution to folks in this age group is advised. Remind them that they should take their time after the massage and take a few deep breaths. The last thing anyone wants is to do a face plant with the floor.

I say this tongue-in-cheek but it's just bad for business. Tell them not to test gravity if they can help it.

It can happen to any of our clients at any age but really we need to be aware of this with our elderly clients.

Session Thirteen
BOOMERANGS

Karma, Golden Rule, what goes around comes around, boomerang effect. However you phrase it, think about it or live your life, I believe their are things that truly do come back to us. Good and bad, the way we treat each other speaks volumes about us and will reflect our true selves.

I have learned that some of the best ways to improve the community's knowledge of you is by being an active part of it on a very real level.

We have a yearly 24 hour relay in town that benefits the Police and community events here in Abington, PA. Organizers for this event look for volunteers for food vendors, musicians and other entertainment and first aid crews. Massage therapy has it's own tent.

Each year I have volunteered for a four hour stint. The kids who run and walk during this 24 hours are so much fun and they also have muscle aches and spasms. They need the attention while they're there. Some of my favorite massage moments are from those relay events. I always come out of there with a huge smile on my face. If you make a good impression, they'll bring back your name or business card to their parents who may in turn call you. Sometimes there are local charities or sponsorships that need support. Gift cards for a particular spa treatment or massage generate a good bit of money for scholarship funds, raffles and different events. I'm not saying that a lot of money needs to go into the community and I'm not saying that you should always give away your services. Far from that. I tire of organizations who tell us to give discounts to everyone and sell packages at a low cost to generate income. Dentists, hair salons, barbers don't do that and neither should we unless you feel it is necessary to help generate additional income or build your clientele list. Once you're in this field for a while, you bring the experience to it and should charge appropriately. Guidelines to use would be similar to the fees charged by other massage offices or spas. You can get a ball park figure for what you should charge. Never charge more than what you are worth and never undercharge your value and experience either.

I was in the field about 5 years when I moved into a new building. I ran an advertisement and press release in the local community. One day a woman called and told me she wanted a massage but that my price was too high. It was perfectly priced within the local community because I had done my checking. She continued to tell me several times that she could get a massage cheaper at "no-name massage office" to which I replied, "If you can get it cheaper and that's what you want to do, then I suggest you call them to make an appointment." There was silence on the other end of the phone. She wanted me to reduce my fees but I had no intention of doing that. I valued my experience and the quality of my work. I think she was shocked. I'm also certain that I don't only want the clients who are looking for a bargain when they should be looking for a quality therapist.

Some of the other ways to improve your visibility is to donate to local teams and organizations, like schools doing plays and need advertisers for their playbills or team jerseys. Sometimes it doesn't generate much in the way of clientele but it's good public relations. So do it sparingly if it doesn't work well for you. We had a teenage girl in our neighborhood pass away from cancer a few years ago and her parents organized a school scholarship fund in her name that was to run for five years. I donated to that. It's a commitment that was important to me. When people see you caring and supporting their efforts, they care more about your business and you as well.

I also suggest joining efforts with a large organization to volunteer using either your massage training or as ancillary personnel. Your efforts don't go unnoticed. It's exposure that is quality and there is little to no cash outlay. It's just dedicating time to a good cause. When I became part of the MS Society's 2 day 30 mile event, I organized spa days at my office with all the proceeds going to my team. All that money goes to research for a cause that I care about. We had a great day of volunteers who truly touched people with their gifts of time and experience.

So always keep things fresh and use all the social media that's out there. Know how the public communicates and jump on board.

Complacency is never good when you run your own business. Keep checking yourself against your business goals that you've set.

Session Fourteen
IN THE BEGINNING

When I began almost 18 years ago, I had no idea what my world would become, how much my clients would become integrated into my life and interestingly how invested in my life they would be.

The clients who retain you as "their therapist" truly value your work, you as a person and anticipate each session because of the good that comes from being massaged.

At the very beginning of this book, I related a story about my massage associate or the owner of the business where I worked and what she told me. She said, "It's not about the money, Cyndi. It's about making them happy and they'll come back."

I am here to tell you that not only do they come back but they also refer others. For years, I have seen this borne out.

It takes a lot to give 100% every time but it's so worth the reward of knowing my clients are really happy and want to share me with their friends and family. I have clients who move away to other states and then return for a massage when they're in town. It is a wonderful thing. You can have that too. That is success in my book. Continue learning, growing from the experiences you have.

Be grateful and kind and always treat the client the way you want to be treated when you receive massage. Find ways to work with people so that your business continues to grow. Have fun. I hope that some of the hints I have given you and the stories I've shared, help you.

Being aware, showing you care, respecting them and you are a success.

Remember, you won't learn this in massage school.

About the Author

My massage career began in 1995 at Pennsylvania Institute of Massage Therapy in Quakertown, PA. With nearly 18 years as a self employed massage therapist I have seen and heard enough to fill a book. So I decided to do just that.

I've worked closely with chiropractors, other massage therapists and physical therapists to gain an even broader view of the body.

Clients can offer great fodder for stories. When I think about all the people I have worked on I realize that I want to share those stories and experiences with other therapists to make their job easier. Schools sometimes graduate students without fully preparing them for what the real massage world is like. We all need a leg up now and then. So I am sharing what I know anecdotally.

I hope that you find the humor in these tips and anecdotes and also in your own experiences with your own clients.

Some of my best stories come from volunteering at local relay events in my township and also through working with the high school kids who play football, soccer and are very active in cheerleading. Getting involved has really expanded my clientele. What a great clientele I have too. They have voted for me in the Philly Hot List and I won 2nd and 3rd places in consecutive years.

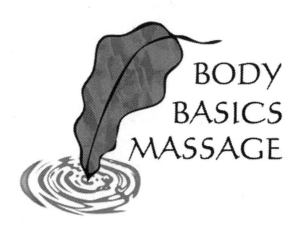

Printed in the United States
By Bookmasters